Dynamic Deployment
A Primer for EMS

John R. Brophy & Dale Loberger

DEDICATION

This book is dedicated to the men and women of EMS past present and future whose efforts to save the lives of their fellow citizens often goes unnoticed.

CONTENTS

FORWARD

Ideas often take time to saturate a market – even the good ideas. It is unfortunate, however, that the best ideas are not always automatically and universally adopted. But change within an organization is often difficult to accept and there is no single approach to ensure success in every situation (Goodman, 1982). Still, in my experience, there are some common qualities that are required for any significant implementation of change. The most necessary forces are a firm understanding of the problem and a determination to implement an effective solution. Through this Primer, the authors attempt to build a foundation for both of these qualities as it relates specifically to achieving efficiency through the dynamic deployment of EMS resources.

The adoption of any technological idea typically follows an "S" shaped curve that describes the gradual adoption of the concept in an early phase which eventually speeds through the majority of a population before slowing again as it reaches saturation. Everett Rogers, a professor of communication studies, popularized this theory in 1962 with his book, "Diffusion of Innovations." A graph demonstrating this performance curve appears below superimposed with a bell shaped curve categorizing individual adopters in his proposed "technology adoption life cycle" (Rogers, 2003).

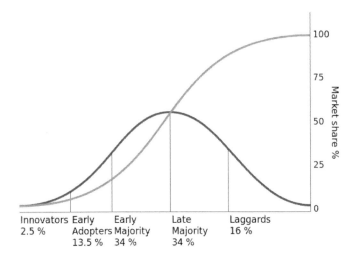

Innovators	Early	Early	Late	Laggards
2.5 %	Adopters	Majority	Majority	16 %
	13.5 %	34 %	34 %	

In the book "Crossing the Chasm," author Geoffery Moore expounds on Rogers ideas by adding a large "crack in the bell curve" that represents a significant cultural chasm that must be crossed before a majority of the population will accept the new idea. Ideas that fail to successfully navigate this gap will also fail to capture a majority of the potential market.

Gartner, Inc. of Stamford, Connecticut, has built a reputation as an information technology research and advisory firm by annually publishing their signature "hype cycle" graphs by industry segment. The basic structure of these graphs start with a technology trigger near the origin of time and visibility followed by a quick rise to the peak of inflated expectations driven by a combination of unrealistic claims by proponents and the hopes of users. The exaggerated peak is inevitably followed by a crash of popularity into the so-called trough of disillusionment. From there, a more realistic set of expectations develop as users may begin to experience positive benefits along the slope of enlightenment before the proven idea plateaus in generally recognized productivity.

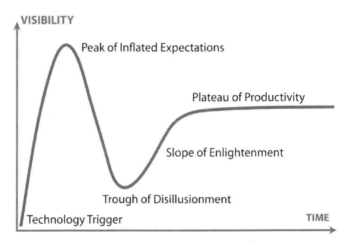

The idea of System Status Management (SSM), brought about by the work of Jack Stout, enjoyed some inflated success early after its advent in the 1980s. Computer processing capabilities, however, along with limited interaction to record systems during the years that followed limited its early success and it fell to a state of general disgrace where many detractors still prefer to think of it. However, many proponents of the early majority have adopted and developed the technology into a working system that delivers real cost savings and improves overall system effectiveness. I believe the technology, as implemented in MARVLIS, is now rising up the slope of enlightenment nearing the plateau of productivity and is attracting a mainstream audience. The final steps in that rise are a general awareness of the actual benefits and how to achieve them. The need for growing that awareness is the reason that this book was conceived. The efficiencies gained by its use in mainstream agencies beyond the initial public utility model organizations seem to vindicate Stout's early vision and research now that the idea is encapsulated in a proven application suite. Ideas are not static entities, but must continue to evolve and incorporate new thoughts. As the iconic American social commentator, Will Rogers said, "Even if you're on the right track, you'll get run over if you just sit there."

Tony Bradshaw

1

STATIC VS. DYNAMIC

Many communities and organizations deploy the same set number of ambulances regardless of hour of day or day of week. Since the configuration does not change, this fixed plan is referred to as a static deployment. This type of plan is very inefficient. There will be times over the course of a day or week when there are far more ambulances available than there are calls requiring them. Some observers might make the argument that because we are dealing with people's lives, the inefficiency is justified as simply a cost of readiness issue. We concur to a point. We need to have sufficient resources to meet the needs. However, a comprehensive analysis of historical call demand can have a positive impact on operations. For best results, it must be done correctly and monitored closely for the inevitable changes that will occur.

On the flip side, with static deployment there will also be times when there will not be enough ambulances for the required call demand. This scenario results in delayed responses and potentially poor patient outcomes. To consider this in lay terms, we all know how frustrating and time consuming it is when we are in a large store and only one or two checkouts are open. We typically go to the store when it was convenient for us. Unfortunately, so did all the others that are now caught in the same bottle-neck that is delaying our quick and efficient check-out. Sometimes we may walk away in disgust or because we simply can't wait any longer. However the majority of us just grind it out and make the best of a bad situation. This is not unlike those people who called 9-1-1 for an ambulance during a time of under deployment. They must spend the extra time waiting because they are forced to make the best of a bad situation.

 In the store example, our time is wasted and the company still gets the sale in spite of their poor planning and resulting slow service. However, in EMS the unnecessary wait can have results far more egregious than the comparatively inconsequential annoyance of spending more time on line in a store.

So how does a discussion about the inefficiencies of a "big-box" store relate to the EMS deployment of ambulances? The point is to illustrate the concept of matching supply with demand in a scenario that many, if not most of us have frequently experienced.

Deployment in EMS is about strategy and tactics. As Sun Tzu wrote centuries ago, "Strategy without tactics is the slowest route to victory." He continued his thought by saying "tactics without strategy is the noise before defeat" (as cited in Kasparov, 2007). Like the check-out lane example, staffing and deploying ambulances requires both strategy and tactics to be successful. Simply staffing and deploying the same amount of units every hour no matter the hour of day or day of the week is a tactic that involves little forethought or strategic thinking. The result is that there will be times of waste (over deployment eating up financial resources) and times of risk (under deployment resulting in extended response times). On the other hand, analyzing historical call demand and building a strategic deployment model that identifies which hours of the day need more and less units will provide a framework from which an efficient (minimal times of waste) and effective (minimal times of risk) schedule can be built and administered. So in short, analysis is the strategy Sun Tzu refers to in this case and how that analysis is interpreted and implemented represents the tactics that follow.

In his work on risk management, Gordon Graham (2004) tells us things that the things that go wrong in life are predictable and predictable is preventable. Dynamic deployment does not "predict" when and where calls will happen. However, when it is effectively utilized it has an eerily accurate ability to forecast the cyclical nature of the human experience as it relates to EMS.

To illustrate, the following graph depicts static deployment against the reality of historical call demand that varies by hour of day and day of week:

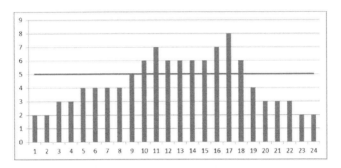

The vertical bars represent the call volume by hour of the day and the horizontal line illustrates the depiction of five ambulances being deployed 24/7. In this depiction of a daily deployment model we see a number of hours where there were far more ambulances than there were calls for service needing them in the early and late hours of the day. In contrast, there are also a number of hours where the bars (calls) tower above the horizontal line (ambulances). During these hours there are insufficient numbers of ambulances to meet the needs of the people calling for them. This common approach results in wasted hours as well as hours where people wait longer for an ambulance because there are not enough available.

A deployment model that is based on historical call demand for each hour of the day and day of the week matches supply and demand. This type of model allows agencies to better utilize their resources and justify

4

requests for increased funding to support increased staffing when necessary. Using the same call demand as depicted above, let's look what happens when we adjust and schedule dynamically based on demand:

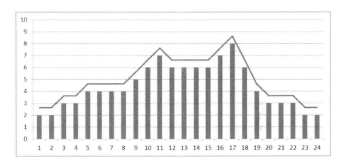

Interestingly, the above dynamic deployment depiction illustrates the same number of ambulance unit hours deployed as the previous plan. Viewing it in this way, we can see there where were enough ambulance hours being scheduled. They were just scheduled at the wrong times in many cases.

Remember these illustrations are just the tip of the iceberg to illustrate the core concept of dynamic versus static deployment. In order to create plans that are more operational analysis and deployment models also need to factor in many variables. Absentee rates, total mission time, lost unit hours for mechanical breakdowns and other inefficiencies top the list. In addition, geographic and contractual constraints must also be considered.

According to Kotler and Caslione (2009) it is important to remember that the decisions a leader makes, especially during turbulent times will have a lasting and significant impact not only on the bottom line but on employees, morale, and even the culture and values that define the company. This is particularly true if the decision undermines the company's fundamentals or fails to meet customers' expectations. We cite their work here as a preface to what follows. In the final analysis, it does not matter if your organization is making deployment adjustments because of a turbulent event such as the loss of a subsidy or contract, or whether it is simply to improve already high-quality service and keep it cutting edge. The important lesson is that the decisions EMS leaders make impact the lives of many, many people. As such these decisions need to be well thought out and promptly acted upon. The development of a strategy to address the issues at hand will provide the foundation. From there the implementation phase of a revised deployment model and a host of other activities will become the tactics that make the strategy possible.

As we proceed, it is important to keep an open mind to ideas with which you are unfamiliar. Ask questions about the ones you are not sure of. And by all means challenge the ones with which you disagree. Just as we believe in the dynamic deployment concepts and the power of predictive software, we also believe these concepts would not exist if people had not challenged the status-quo. An Understanding that an expansion of our knowledge base also expands our horizon of possibilities is at the core of the mindset required to get the most from our study and the application of these concepts (Michaelson and Michaelson, 2010). The importance of asking questions like "why" and "what if" will serve to further clarify and validate these concepts in your own mind. They will also open up new avenues of exploration into a set of next generation concepts that will do nothing but find even better ways to address the ever changing challenges of EMS.

NOTE: Depictions in this chapter assume 1 call equals 1 hour. We will explore the impact of shorter and longer task times in another chapter.

2

FORECASTING TECHNOLOGY

A traditional tabular analysis of historical call data provides an organization with information upon which to make informed decisions about how many unit hours they need to get the job done. It provides a means of forecasting cost and benefit. What it does not provide is the critical "where" aspect.

This spatial component has been the elusive missing piece of the puzzle needed to make SSM work in a highly reliable way. Many agencies either had one System Status Plan (SSP) that was used 24/7/365, 168 SSPs each week that were rotated at the top of the hour, or a homegrown hybrid that fell somewhere between the two. Like the static deployment models, these represented the best thinking so far. These words remind us the future always holds the possibility of additional evidence and better thinking (Adler, 1981). Predictive software as an adjunct to dynamic deployment represents the next leg in our quest for better ways to provide EMS to the public.

The foundation of planning begins by visualizing the future with respect to the present. In terms of EMS resource deployment, those building blocks consist of knowing when and where services will be needed. To further enhance performance knowing the location of resources available and how much area they can cover is essential. Although there are many other considerations that will help refine and improve performance, having the right units at the right places at the right times is the foundation.

We often hear that accidents are random events and that no one can predict the future. And while that statement is superficially true, it also disguises the evidence that recognizable patterns really do exist in human activity (Ying, 2014). Patterns of emergency department usage are certainly no exception (Vieira, 2012). Consider the fact that people have a general affinity to living and working in clusters that share certain socioeconomic, demographic, and geographic similarities with each other (Pedigo, 2011). Studies in the composition of these social groups, as neighborhoods, have shown that predictors exist to subjectively assess community problems (Schieman, 2009). Further, even the perceptions of the community have been shown to impact the level of physical activities and other health determinants (Datar, 2013). Geographic and racial differences also predict whether proactive treatment is sought for preventable diseases (Will, 2014). Neighborhood inequalities including traffic volumes and road design have been demonstrated to directly influence the prevalence of traffic accidents (Morency, 2012). All of this is not to say that random acts do not occur, but rather that events that cause ambulances to be dispatched are far from being totally arbitrary. Recognizing and analyzing data in real-time allows EMS organizations to better deploy and respond.

Still doubt the power of patterns in EMS? Ask almost any group of EMTs or paramedics who have worked the same area for a long time about when and where they expect the calls to come from during their shift. Without much hesitation they will be able to express at least a general idea if not certain likely details. Specific calls that actually occur when or where these paramedics predict do not prove that they have any psychic abilities, but rather that they have developed an awareness of natural local patterns. Most professionals develop an intuitive sense for many patterns in their work. Furthermore, they can often list the criteria that will affect changes in those patterns. These conditions may include weather (Horanont, 2013), community events, holiday traffic patterns, time (Magnusson, 2000), seasonal variations (Mohammadian-Hafshejani, 2014), and even phases of the moon (Walker, 2007). This heuristic approach allows for a quicker, but often more error-prone conclusion than those driven by statistical reality (Myers, 1990). That is not to say that they are invalid, just perhaps that they represent incomplete knowledge.

To further illustrate, a study was done in which hour of day and day of week as well as lunar cycles were considered (Tishkowski & Failes,2008). The conclusion of their research was that "contrary to popular myths, this study did not show fluctuating 9-1-1 EMS call volumes related to full moons..." It further concluded that there was merit to concept of gauging daily pre-hospital ambulance responses by day of the week and month of the year. We found this study to be on-point in two ways. First, it reinforced the weakness of anecdotal conclusions. Second, it reinforced the strength and validity of an evidence based, statistical approach to demand forecasting.

Computers allow us to process vast amounts of data in order to discover consistencies that reveal patterns. As it relates to EMS deployment, querying several years of call history for time-of-day, day-of-week, and season-of-year by location allows us to calculate a probability surface of demand for a future hour and day. This resulting map would not pinpoint the next call, but it will show the relative probability of a call originating from any given location. The temporal breadth and depth of the query will determine the period that the generated surface would represent. Increasing the number of years going back can return a greater number of records. In theory this would typically allow for a more precise forecast. However, past precision does not necessarily equate to future accuracy. For example, in a growing community the population densities will shift and alter patterns of behavior. Selecting a greater number of records from long ago will effectively bias the forecast toward trends in more established neighborhoods at the expense of newer ones. This makes the demand forecasting process very similar to weather forecasts. It is not just a matter of simply averaging as much data as possible; it is refining a query in order to return the most appropriate combination of records to represent trends toward the future. The success of these forecasts will be enhanced with the quality of the actions taken to meet the actual demand as it happens in real-time. This is where science meets art.

Many practitioners compare the demand forecasts to weather forecasts because both use a scientific understanding of the processes involved to project how conditions will continue to evolve. In reality, it is more appropriately described as a form of actuarial science because the demand generation process uses mathematical and statistical methods to assess risk. This risk is expressed through a map as the probability of future requests for service. Demand, therefore, is not represented as likely points where calls will originate, but as a continuum of probability highlighting significant "hot spot" areas where calls are most likely to occur. Refining these areas leverages the "art" of the actuarial process to achieve the most actionable information. Once it is mastered, the MARVLIS Demand Monitor automates the forecasting procedure as a scheduled system process employing SQL queries and modelling the results spatially through ArcGIS, a product of Esri, Inc. This allows it to be visualized on a map. Because the process is automated, it can be executed several times each hour to give an accurate view of future demand as each work shift progresses. Internal studies at BCS, Inc. have shown that properly modeled demand typically highlights hot spots consisting collectively of little more than 10-15% of the total geography of the service area. This is significant because these isolated areas contain nearly 80% of the actual incoming calls. Knowing where and when to expect future calls gives any service an advantage in addressing those calls quickly and safely by pre-positioning vehicles closer to the calls before the phone is even dialed.

Successful dynamic deployment also requires dispatchers to know the real-time locations of all resources. Many agencies have formal Automated Vehicle Location (AVL) applications to track and monitor their fleets. The data collected often includes a vehicle identifier with a date/time stamp of when the record was collected along with the vehicle position (in longitude/latitude), the vehicle speed, and its direction of travel. Sometimes additional vehicle telemetry data is collected for fleet maintenance, fuel economy or other purposes. Even without a formal AVL database, the system can still dynamically dispatch resources if a minimum data set of an identifier, date/time stamp, and position is reported. The missing history of speed and heading data, however, will limit advanced network modeling capabilities.

Traditionally, vehicle assignments were made by referencing a primary service zone, sometimes referred to as a "first due" area. In this case, vehicle assignment was made based on a projected, rather than a verified, vehicle location. Before wireless connectivity was available directly to GPS units within the vehicle, ambulance positions were assumed to be tied to their last known status in the CAD. For instance, an ambulance was considered to be physically located at the hospital as long as the CAD reflects that particular status for a vehicle. It remained mapped to that point until the status was changed to reflect that it was either en-route to a particular station or had arrived at an assigned post. Instantaneously, the position of that vehicle was updated from the hospital to the station even though it was actually traveling somewhere between these known locations for some time. Lacking dynamic mapping capabilities, call assignments were never guaranteed to be made to the actual closest vehicle. If a unit had an available status it was assumed to be within its primary service area. This process, while crude, was easy to implement.

GPS reporting of vehicle position in near real-time along with the ability to calculate a dynamic service area surrounding a moving vehicle changed the basic rules. Response zones no longer needed to be fixed areas surrounding a base assignment theoretically covering every possible location. Instead, animated maps become fluid representations of a unit's actual coverage within a defined response time. Consequently, response zones no longer need to represent the entire service area. Instead they can now represent the system's current ability to respond within specific time parameters more precisely.

As vehicles continue to travel, their dynamic service area representation will change immediately with each new GPS position report. The shape of these individual response zones change quickly in relation to the street configuration around each vehicle earning them descriptive nicknames such as "blob" or "amoeba." As additional vehicles become available, their dynamic service area representations are automatically added to the map. Likewise, as units become unavailable, their service area representations disappear from the overall system map. At any given point in time, the map represents the agency's ability to meet service time objectives. When the dynamic service areas cover the highest demand probabilities the likelihood of meeting response time goals in a safe and efficient manner is increased.

Systems that have extensive AVL databases, including both speed and direction, can take the network modeling capabilities even further to achieve a greater degree of accuracy in routing and the estimation of travel times. The general assumption that ambulances consistently travel at posted speed limits is simplistic. At certain times they will be able to safely travel faster while other times they will be consistently delayed even using lights and sirens. Still most routing algorithms only model travel at posted rates for every road segment and even the more advanced applications model heavy traffic in real time at the average rate for vehicles in that direction. Emergency vehicles can avoid traffic delays by using road shoulders to bypass traffic or even utilize opposing traffic lanes. To model these unique travel patterns, it is your own past fleet data that is most valuable.

With a little intuition of the traffic pattern periods throughout each day and week, your AVL data can be queried to retrieve the speeds by location and direction of travel during these various identified periods to model more realistic travel impedances. To refine the values even further, the records queried for the impedance calculations can be limited to only include certain response codes. For instance, to model how quickly an Advanced Life Support (ALS) team can arrive at a scene when dispatched at 0800 on a summer Tuesday morning, the AVL database can be queried for only "code 3" responses during a normal morning weekday rush period when school is not in session. This form of impedance calculation develops an average speed specific to emergency response vehicles based on any identified traffic period. The morning "rush hour" around a significant city will be very different from the evening "drive home" pattern. The higher impedance to travel is always heading with traffic while travel against that traffic is typically much easier. Real-time traffic can be helpful in knowing about specific unique roadway situations, but it is currently of limited value in EMS. Once that data becomes standardized in content and format, it will likely offer more value in travel estimates. Dispatchers already note that the MARVLIS Impedance Monitor provides travel estimates that are within seconds of actual experienced times when their own history is used in learning traffic impedances.

Dynamic deployment technology also extends beyond the dispatch center into the vehicle by allowing crews to not only receive route recommendations on their laptops or tablets within the ambulance, but it can allow crews to update their CAD status at the press of a button rather than relaying the change through radio traffic to a dispatcher for entry to the CAD. A centralized routing process also simplifies updates of planned construction projects or major accidents that will affect routing times without the data having to chase ambulances for inclusion with local calculations. The centralized MARVLIS Server also facilitates browser based map views of the overall system including all of the tracked vehicles and active incidents for administrative situational reporting using MARVLIS Sitrep Global. This personal web experience allows each user to customize a map display suited to their specific needs.

Together with a staffing model that balances the historical call demand, budgetary, contractual, and human resource considerations, the dynamic forecasting and tracking software represents the next generation in the evolution of EMS deployment.

3

ANALYZING YOUR SYSTEM

Triage in the field has been around since the days of
Napoleon when it is believed his surgeon Baron
Dominique-Jean Larrey (1766–1842) first developed the
concepts of both an ambulance corps and a field triage
system (Balane, 2011). Why do we mention this at the
top of a chapter on analyzing your system? There are
two reasons. First, it is to illustrate that pre-hospital
emergency medical care has been, and always will be, in
an evolutionary state. The second reason is to set the
stage for this chapter using one of the key concepts of
triage - start where you stand.

An analysis of your EMS deployment plan starts with
your system in its current state. No matter the findings
as they relate to dynamic deployment, every EMS
system has opportunities for improvement. While we
are presenting some nationally accepted best practices,
one thing we have learned over the years is that "if you
have seen one EMS system, you have seen one EMS
system." Meaning there is no "one-size-fits-all"

approach to dynamic deployment just as there is no singular solution to anything else we do in EMS.

There are lots of variables like specific contractual requirements, budgetary constraints, political implications, and so forth. All of which must be considered, but we believe there is a logical process to the evaluation. The first step being to determine if there are sufficient resources to provide the services required or if there are any opportunities for savings. In short, the analysis is about seeing where you stand in relation to where you need to be, or where you would ultimately like to be.

Conducting a demand analysis is an essential element to determine how many units are needed at what hours of the day and days of the week. To determine this we need to look at the historical call volume, compare it to the existing schedule, and address the findings.

An EMS organization must look at deployment from a variety of perspectives to accomplish their responsibilities. As such we need to calculate the total number of units needed in an hour, for an entire day, week, pay-period, month, and year. To do this, we need to start with the smallest common piece of these measurement intervals. According to Rene Descartes, a 17th Century mathematician and philosopher (as cited in Van Doren, 1991) when a problem seems too big and complicated, break it down into small problems. As such, let us begin our exploration of calculus as it relates to EMS deployment.

When looking at a week's historical call demand we must first break it down into the 168 hours of the week so that we can build an hour-by-hour demand model. It is important to keep this figure in mind as we talk about these concepts throughout the chapter. We will be looking at each hour of the day, by day of the week, and conducting our calculations for each as we work through the process. From there we can build the hour by hour staffing models we need for the weekly schedule. This will roll-up into the larger measurements of unit hours the people around us need as well. The key is getting each hour correct so that everything that builds off of it will be sound.

There are a number of ways to determine the demand from which to build an EMS deployment schedule. Any one of them, however, requires a statistically valid data sample size to assure that no matter which method of calculation is used, it will be valid. From our research and application, we have found that 20 weeks of call data is a reasonable and practical beginning point for accurate forecasting calculations. Therefore, for purposes of our studies, we will base all of our calculations on that premise.

As mentioned at the top of this discussion, there are a number of ways to look at the data with respect to deployment decisions. To be better prepared to determine which method best fits a particular organization's needs, it is important to understand what those needs are and what they represent. This understanding will allow for informed decisions relative to balancing performance against the cost of readiness.

Three common ways are to base the demand analysis are on average volume, average high volume, or average peak volume.

Average Volume is perhaps the simplest of the calculations as it simply takes the total volume for each hour and divides it by the total number of hours included in the sample. To illustrate, we will use one hour of the week. Total all of the calls for the 20 week period within that hour and divide that number by 20.

2	2	3	3	2	5	0	5	7	4	2	3	2	5	0	5	3	3	2	3

The record above represents the number of calls during the same hour for each of 20 consecutive weeks. In this example, there were a total of 61 calls over the 20 week period for the hour selected. This example would produce an **Average** of 3.05 calls on that hour during those days.

Using this model we could make the decision to staff three (3) units for this particular hour. It seems Pretty straight forward, but here is the catch. Doing so would only provide us with a reliability factor of about 70%.

This is because deploying 3 units would only be sufficient in 14 of the 20 weeks.

Before we get caught-up on the reliability factor for average, let's take a look at the reliability factors for the other means of analyzing demand as a means of comparison.

Average High is the average of the highest number of calls in each set of four consecutive weeks. So, using the same 20 week period lets now look at Average High.

2	2	**3**	3
2	**5**	0	5
7	4	2	3
2	5	0	**5**
3	**3**	2	3

The above represents five sets of four consecutive weeks each with the high for each set in **bold**.

In this case we would take the average of 3, 5, 7, 5, and 3. Doing so gives us an **Average High** of 4.60 calls per hour.

If we were to staff for average high we would achieve a reliability factor of 75% to 90% depending which way we decided to round the partial unit.

Average Peak is the average of the peak (highest) volume in the first 10 weeks (weeks 1-10) and the peak (highest) volume in the second 10 weeks (weeks 11-20). Once again using the above 20 weeks, let's look at Average Peak.

2	2	3	3	2	5	0	5	**7**	4
2	3	2	**5**	0	5	3	3	2	3

In this case we would take the average of 7 and 5. This would give us an average peak volume of 6 calls in the hour or the period studied.

Staffing to average peak in this case would produce a reliability factor of 95%.

So, with the choice of Average Volume of 3.05 calls, an Average High Volume of 4.60 and an Average Peak volume of 6, which do we choose as the base for our deployment? Before answering that question let's look a little deeper into what impact staffing to each of these levels will have on availability, cost, and ultimately performance.

According to Gridley (2001) using average you can expect to have enough units to make 50% response compliance. With average high that expectation would be 75% and using average peak it would be 90%. But the question is which foundation is most appropriate for your model. We now know the answer depends on a number of the factors previously discussed.

Obviously better reliability and contractual compliance are essential. But let's take a look at the cost of readiness.

Looking first at the hour from our example above, let's compare the cost of deployment for just that one hour out of 168 each week and compare based on Average, Average High, and Average Peak. For this calculation, we need to know the cost of a deployed unit hour. For the purposes of discussion, we will use $75 as that cost.

To deploy at Average would cost us $228.75 per hour ($75 x 3.05), while Average High would cost $345 per hour ($75 x 4.6) and Average Peak would run our cost up to $450 per hour ($75 x 6). And remember this is just for the one hour in our example. The following is a comparative annual cost for just this one hour over the course of the entire year (52 Weeks).

Average	Average High	Average Peak
$11,895	$17,940.0	$23,400

As we know from our discussions of static and dynamic deployment, each hour of the day and day of the week will be different. With That said, we will assume Average, Average High, and Average Peak worked out to be 3.05, 4.6, and 6 respectively (same as it did for our calculation above) just for the purposes of illustration of the calculations. Using those numbers and our same $75 cost per unit hour here is the annual cost difference.

Average	Average High	Average Peak
$1,998,360	$3,013,920	$3,931,200

As we see from the example above, there is a clearly defined cost to the readiness and reliability that must be considered when building a schedule. The lesson here is that there is a way to calculate how to build a schedule that meets goals and constraints. With this information EMS leadership can make informed decisions about deployment. These decisions can be backed up with data about cost and projections of reliability.

In summary, a dynamic system requires a strong foundation based on facts. To be successful, EMS leaders must understand what the numbers mean and how they impact operations. EMS has come a long way since the ambulance corps of Napoleon's era. What we have managed to accomplish to this point is in large part because of our collective creativity and a desire to do better for tomorrow than we did yesterday. Looking critically at what we do and always seeking to improve is a legacy for which EMS can be proud.

4

UNDERSTANDING YOUR METRICS

It has been said, and repeated by many, that "you can't manage what you don't measure." We're not sure who first said it but it has been accepted as a valid point in many circles. At this juncture we would like to propose a modification to it. So here goes... "Without measuring it we can't manage it well." This modification to the concept is based on our experience and observations over time. The trick, however, is in knowing exactly what needs to be managed and how to measure it. Conversely, just because something is easy to measure doesn't necessarily make it a management objective.

Since different things are important to different people the question becomes what to measure. Chute times, response times, Time on Task (TOT), Unit Hour Utilization (UHU), and so many other metrics compete for attention. To complicate matters even further, results of the same metric will often have different meanings to different people. For example, a higher UHU looks great to finance, but operations feels the stress of staff working harder. On the flip side, a lower

UHU stresses the budget while the staff feels some relief.

Why do we mention this? To illustrate that while we profess the need to measure what we do in EMS, we also need to remember that these numbers almost always involve people's lives, either of our staff or the public in general. In short, the measurement is easy, it's the interpretation of the measures and to the actions we make to sustain a positive direction in the organization that is more of a challenge. This is the crossroads of science and art.

Let's take a look at some common measurements and why they are important:

Unit Hour Utilization (UHU) is the percentage of time that fully staffed and equipped units are actually on calls. This percentage would be marked from time of dispatch until time available either for posting or the next call. The formula being calls/unit hours = UHU. For example, let's look at an agency that had 30 calls in a day with each taking one hour to complete. If the agency had a deployment of 100 unit hours the UHU for that day would be 0.30.

Notice that we qualified the formula by saying expressing the assumption that each call took an hour. Often times UHU is simply measured based on the premise that one call takes one hour to complete. This assumption is fine in theory and works in practice when one call routinely takes an actual hour. However, before using the academic and theoretical assumption, you should investigate the records in your Computer Aided Dispatch (CAD) database to determine your actual time on task (sometimes referred to as total mission time) based on your own call history. If it is anything other than 60 minutes, you need to factor it appropriately into the equation.

We will delve further into this topic after we fully define time on task and illustrate it using the same example of 30 calls and 100 unit hours as above, but with different time on task averages.

Time on Task (TOT) sometimes referred to a Total Mission Time (TMT) is measured from dispatch through the completion of a call. TOT is an important measurement with respect to UHU and has an impact on both the bottom line and operational effectiveness.

If a TOT was 60 minutes then the hour-to-call ratio of one-to-one illustrated above would hold true. But since the TOT is either more or less than a precise 60 minutes, the actual value needs to be taken into consideration when calculating UHU or anything else that uses TOT as part of the equation.

Let's look at the above calculation when TOT is actually 66 minutes. To do so we need to divide 66 minutes by 60. This gives us a factor of 1.1 to represent TOT. In so doing we find that 30 calls at 66 minutes TOT is the equivalent of 33 hours of utilization. So, 33 hours utilization/100 unit hours deployed equals 0.33 UHU. As you can see the UHU increased because the amount of time it took to complete each call increased. At the same time the total number of unit hours deployed remained the same.

On the flip side, suppose the TOT is 54 minutes. In this case the TOT factor would be established by dividing 54 minutes by 60. This gives us a factor of .9 to represent TOT. This results in a UHU of .27 because each call takes less than an hour to complete. So whether the TOT is greater than or less than 60 minutes factoring the equation accordingly will impact UHU.

Lost Unit Hours (LUH) include the hours that were scheduled, but are for some reason not available for calls. This includes anything that reduces the total unit hours such as an employee calling out sick or starting a shift late. But let's not pin the blame for lost unit hours entirely on the staff. Rather than placing blame at all it is more beneficial to look for the causes of lost unit hours. Doing so will allow us to fix them. The following list is not all inclusive, but is representative of some of the common causes of lost unit hours:

1.   Inefficient shift change

2.   Mechanical failure

3.   Turn-around times

4. Employee's calling out sick

5. Tardiness

6. Unfilled shifts (open positions, vacations, etc.)

Lost unit hours impact operations greatly and must be monitored and managed to achieve success. Consider the UHU calculations discussed earlier. Lost unit hours must be deducted from the total scheduled hours thereby driving up the UHU from a perspective of crew workload. Increasing the UHU shows a direct negative impact on crews for these LUH. As a result, crews are working harder and response times are suffering because there are less effective unit hours while deployed costs remain the same. Effectively, we are paying the same price, but stressing our people and achieving a lower overall quality.

Effective Unit Hours (EUH) are the hours that remain after all of the inefficiencies of lost unit hours are subtracted from the scheduled hours. To put it a formula:

scheduled hours – lost unit hours = effective unit hours

Knowing effective unit hours is important. It impacts the above calculations. To get a more precise depiction of UHU the equation would divide the factored number of calls by the effective unit hours. To illustrate, suppose the 66 minute TOT was measured against 92 hours of deployment instead of 100. The result would be a .36 UHU.

Other metrics to consider include fractile response times, average response times, unloaded miles driven, and post moves to name a few.

When implementing a dynamic deployment system with predictive software both fractile and average response times should improve. Fractile improvement represents the increased reliability of the system to achieve more timely responses. Average response time represents shorter responses, which means less time and distance (often under lights and sirens) driven from dispatch to on-scene. This shorter emergency response distance equates to improved safety for personnel and the public alike.

Post moves and unloaded miles, while non-traditional metrics, are listed because they impact both employee morale and the bottom line. It is important to establish your baseline for both before implementation. For best results they must be continually monitored going forward with adjustments made to operations as needed. Staff members, especially those who do not understand or embrace the dynamic deployment concept, often perceive that they are moving posts more often and driving more miles. Sometimes they will support their beliefs through specific anecdotes. However, by tracking these metrics you can show that this does not occur or take appropriate action if it does.

Paramedics and EMTs are accustomed to evidence-based practice, so it is important that you have tangible data to share with your people to help bridge the gap between perception and reality.

These "non-traditional" metrics were added to reinforce the importance of the third, and often overlooked, piece of the Quality Unit Hour Concept (Stout, 2005). The piece we are referring to is "employee wellbeing". By design, employee wellbeing must be balanced with patient care and financial stability for best results. Under-estimating the value of your employees' morale is a significant detriment to successful system implementation.

By monitoring and managing post moves and unloaded miles, EMS organizations can provide for a safer work environment for everyone. Fewer post moves and less overall miles driven equate to more "down time" for your staff. As a result, "workload" is reduced by requiring less driving between calls.

The organization saves as well, less miles driven equates to direct cost savings in fuel and maintenance.

Finally, the patient also benefits because crews are available at the times and places they are needed.

These two "non-traditional" metrics are just the tip of the iceberg. They are a reminder not to be limited in our thinking. Watch your metrics, but listen to your people and your customers. Find out what is important to them and create a new metric to measure it. It has been said that the sky is the limit. But if that is the case then why are there footprints on the moon? Point being, don't be limited by current thinking.

In retrospect, the three letter abbreviation, SSM, has become a four letter word to some. This perception is largely due to the fact that these (and other) non-traditional metrics have not previously been considered. As a result the employee wellness component did not receive enough attention in the core system design and everyone suffered.

Finally, the development of forecasting software has demonstrated its ability to create more effective dynamic posting operations. This technological advance has provided yet another tool that was not available in the original SSM toolbox. This more efficient design is to EMS what fuel injectors are to automobiles - a newer and more effective technology designed as an enhancement.

5

IMPLEMENTATION AND CHANGE

Since the late 1960's Emergency Medical Services (EMS) has grown and emerged into a profession that has seen more improvements in out-of-hospital care than in all prior millennia (Brennan and Krohmer, 2006). During this time the public has become both more reliant on and more educated about EMS. Their expectations are high, as they should be. They demand accountability and ask questions when they believe we have missed the mark. They demand accountability more now than ever before. As such we must continually strive for better ways to provide our services

In its simplest form, change has three phases – the current state, the state of transition, and the desired state. The first and last phases are easy compared to the state of transition. The first is where we are and the last is where we want to be. The state of transition, as Conner (1992) puts it is a state that is uncomfortable as "no one likes existing in a state of limbo because the in-between periods in our lives are filled with instability, conflict, and high stress". It is because of this that leaders must understand change and the reactions people have to it so that they can account for it in their planning and execution of the achievement of the desired result.

Let's take a look now at some of the reasons people resist change. There are many reasons for sure, but for purposes of our conversation we are going to rely upon a list put forth by Professor Gary Yukl in his text *Leadership in Organizations*:

1. Lack of trust

2. Belief that the change is unnecessary

3. Belief that the change is not feasible

4. Economic threats

5. Relative high costs

6. Fear of personal failure

7. Loss of status and power

8. Threat to values and ideals

9. Resentment of interference

Looking over this list we see a few items that will likely crop up when implementing a dynamic deployment system. We would guess, if not bet, that each one of us has either seen or felt one or more of these resistances to change in some aspect of our lives.

Seeing it in others is one thing, but reality is that the cases in which we felt it reinforce the fact that Yukl (2006) is correct that these reactions to change are not simply academic.

Knowing and having even experienced some, if not most of these resistances allows leaders to be better prepared to account for them when embarking on a mission of change. Unfortunately no matter how well we prepare the resistance will still be there, but that does not excuse us from doing so, in fact it requires us to so that we can minimize the gap between the current status and the envisioned or desired status.

In looking at this list we see five key elements of leadership that must be employed when leading change:

1. Building and sustaining trust

2. Actively listening to the people around you

3. Actively communicating the vision and the why (reasons for change) behind the what (change itself)

4. Knowing and understanding your people

5. Knowing your organization and your industry

In short, this list boils down to the fact that a leader must do their homework and take the steps necessary to achieve the desired result with the least amount of disruption during the transition.

We provided this brief look at change and the reactions to it as yet another primer for EMS leaders considering a transition from static to dynamic deployment. While brief, we felt hitting some high points and taking the time to remind ourselves that resistance to change is part of life was a worthwhile endeavor. No matter how well intentioned and well planned a change is there will always be resistance. Accepting this reality allows the EMS leader to better navigate the change process.

When transitioning from static to dynamic deployment almost every area of the organization will be impacted. As such, we would like to key in on some common areas affected with thoughts to consider.

Dispatch will be transitioning from a static approach that is clearly defined to one in which there are more variables and more right ways to do it than wrong. There will no longer be an absolute way to post three ambulances versus four. They will be transitioning from one-directional "checkers" to multi-directional "chess". The ability to think strategically will be paramount. The ability to see the whole board and look a few more moves ahead will serve them well.

Field personnel will often question post moves based on early anecdotes. They will perceive more movement from post to post, which initially may be the case. But will resolve in time. This is why it is vitally important that the metrics we discussed be monitored. We need to keep the hiccups of implementation to a minimum and be responsive to the concerns of the field staff. In fairness, they will likely be feeling the most transition anxiety until the dust settles.

Often the focus of an implementation is on dispatch, but field personnel must be included from the start in any implementation. Input on where to add or remove posts is one example of where their expertise is invaluable. The data in dispatch may show that there are "hot spots" from time to time in areas we don't have posts. Connecting with field operations and soliciting their suggestions for posts that are safe and comfortable in a given geographic area will have significant positive downstream impact.

Since dynamic posting often involves more time in the vehicles and less time in fixed stations consideration must be given to the level of UHU expected. For example, crews that can come back to a static station may find a higher UHU acceptable because they can sit in a chair or on a couch and watch TV in between calls. But crews who spend less time in their stations due to dynamic deployment posting will be less tolerant. As such, when designing your system you may need to budget a lower UHU (less TOT per shift) to address physical and emotional fatigue of your people.

We know a lower UHU as mentioned above impacts the bottom line, but when implemented successfully a dynamic system will provide offsets to balance the books. For example, in one implementation we worked on the organization realized a reduction of over 1600 unloaded miles driven per week. Doing the math on the savings in fuel and maintenance costs this type of added efficiency can help the bottom line while simultaneously allowing room for a lower UHU. Again, it is about monitoring, measuring, and adjusting or sustaining then repeating the same cycle.

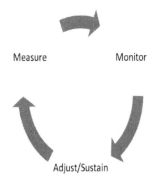

Measure   Monitor

Adjust/Sustain

Another aspect of leading change from a static to a dynamic system is addressing the change anxiety and resistance that may be experienced by government officials and the public. It is vital that they are educated about and included in the process early on and throughout. They will have some of the same questions your staff did and likely a few more. Take the time to educate them and take the time to listen to them. We don't know where the next great idea will come from.

Some agencies we have worked with have had great success in this area. When key members of the public understood both the "what" and the "why" they became surrogate advocates. Some even developed partnerships that allowed for designated parking spaces in which to post and staff use of their facilities while at post.

After Joan Lunden left Good Morning America (GMA) she embarked on a journey of finding and creating her new normal. Among her accomplishments since leaving GMA was a book she wrote called *A Bend in the Road Is Not the End of the Road* (1998). It is about dealing with change and some principles she discovered and used along her journey of change. In her book she writes "We cannot avoid change. It is the one constant in our lives, yet it produces the greatest amount of fear."

A successful implementation of a dynamic deployment system requires the coordination of a variety of sometimes competing priorities. While sound in the science it is the art component that each agency must also master with respect to the nuances of both the system and the community. Most importantly, at its core making such a transition is an exercise in change leadership. Don't let a fear of change deter you. Take the time to help those less comfortable with change understand what is going on. Doing so will help turn the energy created by their fears into a positive force in support of your efforts to improve performance.

According to Adler (1981) the judgment that something is good or bad – or better or worse than something else – is one we make every day, often many times a day. As the contemporary leaders of EMS we owe it to our predecessors who pioneered EMS. They have left a legacy and entrusted us with its future to continue that pioneering spirit in how we carry the torch they have passed to us. We must, as they did, look for new ad better ways to do things. We must realize that what works today can always be better and may not work as well, or at all in the future.

REFERENCES AND RESOURCES

Adler, M. J. (1981). *Six Great Ideas*. New York, NY: Touchstone.

Balane, F.G. (2011) *A Brief History of Triage*. Retrieved from http://www.scribd.com/doc/62923941/A-Brief-History-of-Triage on July 5, 2014

Brennan, J. A., & Krohmer J. R. (Eds.). (2006). *Principles of EMS Systems*. Sudbury, Massachusetts: Jones and Bartlett Publishers.

Brophy, J. R. (2014) *21st Century Leadership*. Charleston, SC: Create Space.

Datar, A., Nicosia, N., & Shier, V. (2013). Parent Perceptions of Neighborhood Safety and Children's Physical Activity, Sedentary Behavior, and Obesity: Evidence from a National Longitudinal Study. *American Journal of Epidemiology*, *177*(10), 1065-1073.

Goodman, P. (1982). *Change in Organizations: New perspectives on theory and research and practice*. San Francisco: Jossey-Bass Inc.

Graham, G. (2004). Managing the Risky Business of EMS. *In Proceedings from the EMS Today Conference & Exposition*. Salt Lake City, UT: Elsevier.

Gridley, T. S. (2001, June 10) *Understanding Demand and Building a Demand Analysis*. Lecture presented as

part of a System Status Management Basic and
Advanced Skills-Building Interactive Workshop.
Sheraton Country Square Hotel. Atlanta, Georgia.

Horanont, T., Phithakkitnukoon, S., Leong, T., Sekimoto,
Y., & Shibasaki, R. (2013). Weather effects on the
patterns of people's everyday activities: A study using
GPS traces of mobile phone users. *PLoS ONE, 8*(12), 1-
14.

Hubbard, D. (2004) Three Levels of
Knowledge[Foreward]. In *If Disney Ran Your Hospital: 9
1/2 Things You Would Do Differently* (pp. 1-2).
Bozeman, MT: Second River Healthcare Press.

Kasparov, G. (2007). *How Life Imitates Chess*. New York,
NY: Bloomsbury.

Kotler, P., & Caslione, J. A. (2009). *Chaotics: The
Business of Managing and Marketing in the Age of
Turbulence*. New York, NY: AMACOM.

Magnusson, M. (2000). Discovering hidden time
patterns in behavior: T-patterns and their detection.
Behavior Research Methods, Instruments, & Computers,
32(I), 93-110.

Michaelson, G.A. and Michaelson, S. (2010). *Sun Tzu –
The Art of War for Managers.* Avon, Massachusetts:
Adams Media.

Mohammadian-Hafshejani, A., Sarrafzadegan, N.,
Hosseini, S., Baradaran, H., Roohafza, H., Sadeghi, M., &
Asadi-Lari, M. (2014). Seasonal pattern in admissions

and mortality from acute myocardial infarction in elderly patients in Isfahan, Iran. *ARYA Atherosclerosis, 10*(1), 46-55.

Moore, G. (2002). *Crossing the chasm: Marketing and selling high-tech products to mainstream customers.* New York: Harper Collins.

Morency, P., Gauvin, L., Plante, C., Fornier, M., & Morency, C. (2012). Neighborhood Social Inequalities in Road Traffic Injuries: The Influence of Traffic Volume and Road Design. *American Journal of Public Health, 102*(6), 1112-1119.

Myers, D. G. (1990) *Exploring Psychology.* New York, New York. Worth Publishers, Inc.

Pedigo, A., Seaver, W. & Odoi, A. (2011). Identifying Unique Neighborhood Characteristics to Guide Health Planning for Stroke and Heart Attack: Fuzzy Cluster and Discriminant Analyses Approaches. *PLoS ONE, 6*(7), 1-11.

Rogers, E. (2003). *The diffusion of innovations.* Fifth edition. New York: The Free Press.

Schieman, S. (2009). Residential Stability, Neighborhood Racial Composition, and the Subjective Assessment of Neighborhood Problems Among Older Adults. *Sociological Quarterly, 50*(4), 608-632.

Stout Solutions, LLC (2005) *High Performance EMS Education Series, Level II-C.* Midlothian, VA. Stout Solutions, LLC.

Tishkowski, K., Failes, L., Little, R., Myers, S., & Impens, A. (2008) Relationships of Daily 9-1-1 Emergency Medical Service (EMS) Responses to Lunar Cycles, Holidays, Days of the Week, Months of the Year, and Daily Precipitation. Mobile Medical Response, Saginaw Michigan., Oakwood Healthcare System, Michigan., ER-One, Livonia, Michigan., & University of Michigan, Ann Arbor, Michigan.

United States Department of Agriculture (2013). *Firefighter Math*. Retrieved 11/17/2013 from http://training.nwcg.gov/courses/ffm.

Van Doren, C. (1991). *A History of Knowledge: Past, Present, and Future*. New York: Ballantine Books.

Vieira, V., Weinberg, J., & Webster, T. (2012). Individual-level space-time analyses of emergency department data using generalized additive modeling. *BMC Public Health*, *12*(1), 687-695.

Walker, T., Macfarlane, T., & McGarry, G. (2007). The epidemiology and chronobiology of epistaxis: an investigation of Scottish hospital admissions 1995–2004. *Clinical Otolaryngology*, 32(5), 361-365.
Will, J., Nwaise, I., Schieb, L., & Yuna, Z. (2014). Geographic and Racial Patterns of Preventable Hospitalizations for Hypertension: Medicare Beneficiaries, 2004-2009. *Public Health Reports, 129*(1), 8-18.

Ying, J., Lee, W., Tseng, V. (2014). Mining Geographic-Temporal-Semantic Patterns in Trajectories for Location Prediction. *ACM Transactions on Intelligent Systems & Technology*, 5(1), 1-33.

Yukl, G. (2006). Leadership in Organizations. Upper Saddle River, NJ: Pearson Prentice Hall.

ABOUT THE AUTHORS

John R. Brophy has been in EMS for over 30 years. He has experience in a variety of service delivery models and has experience from provider through director in both field and dispatch operations. His experience with dynamic deployment includes system analysis, implementation, and performance improvement. He has presented dynamic deployment concepts locally to agencies around the country and at the national conference level. He is the author of numerous articles in EMS trade journals as well as three other books – Leadership Essentials for Emergency Medical Services, 21st Century Leadership, and Reflections, A leadership Anthology.

Dale Loberger has been analyzing spatial data and patterns using GIS for over 30 years and has been recognized as both a GIS Professional by the GIS Certification Institute and an ArcGIS Certified Desktop Professional by Esri. His introduction to fire suppression was also over three decades ago when he fought forest fires and studied their behavior. While his career has included many aspects of GIS technology, his fascination with public safety brought him back to the fire service where he now serves as a Lieutenant and EMT. Along with his experience, he brings a passion to improve both the efficiency and efficacy of EMS operations through his work at Bradshaw Consulting Services. Social media serves as a primary engagement for him on the topic of High Performance EMS.

FOR FURTHER INFORMATION

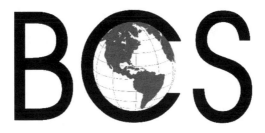

For further information about predictive software applications including MARVLIS please contact BCS at 803-641-0960 or visit www.bcs-gis.com.

For further information on system demand analysis contact John R. Brophy at brophyjohnr@aol.cm.

Made in the USA
San Bernardino, CA
26 March 2015